THE CANNABIS OIL GUIDE

Various Disease Treatments

Using Cannabis Oil

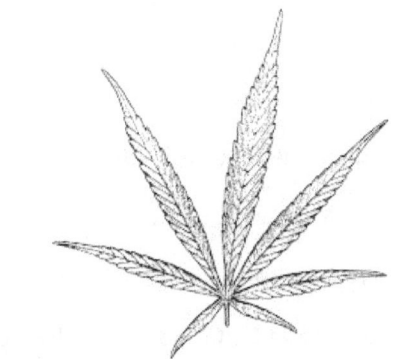

By Martin Pals

Table of content

Introduction ....

    The Sativa Plant ....

    Components of Cannabis Oil ....

How to Obtain and Use Cannabis ....

Cannabis Oil ....

Extracting the Cannabis Oil ....

The importance of Cannabis Oil ....

10 Health treatments using Cannabis Oil ....

    2. Appetite and Obesity ....

    3. Asthma ....

    4. Heart Health ....

    5. Pain Relief ....

    6. Cancer ....

    7. Skin Protection ....

    10. Other Potential Benefits of the Cannabis oil ....

        Headaches and Migraines: ....

The United States' laws on the Cannabis Oil ....

The Difference between the Cannabis oil and Hemp oil ....

Word of Caution ....

Conclusion ....

Introduction

For some time, the medical industry has sought alter-natives in the treatment of certain ailments. This is be- cause of the persistence of some health conditions even after some drugs have been taken. A lot of ailments have proven stubborn hence the search for alternative me-dication.

As technology has evolved, research into the medical world has increased astronomically with the limelight being shown towards the use of natural herbs.

Among such herbs is cannabis oil, which is derived from the Sativa plant. Cannabis is a naturally growing herb that has been used for thousands of years to treat different health conditions. It's also used in making perfumes, soaps, candles, and some other foods and supplements.

Cannabis is a very powerful oil with the ability to treat numerous health conditions, and only small amounts are needed for it to have a powerful effect on the body and mind—hence it is termed a wonder plant. Though serious research is still ongoing, there have been some success stories on the ability of the oil to treat diverse problems.

The Sativa Plant

Cannabis oil can be traced back to the Sativa plant, which is most commonly bred for its potent, sticky glands that are known as trichomes which are a powerful constituent of the oil and which is responsible for its ability in treating many sicknesses. These trichomes are found to contain high amounts of **tetrahydrocannabinol** (generally known as **THC**), which is the cannabinoid most known for its psychoactive properties and therapeutic usefulness.

Due to concerns about the dangers of marijuana abuse in different countries of the world, the sales and movement of this plant were banned for medicinal use in the United States and many other countries in the 1930s and 1940s. Hence it became illegal to be sold or used during this time. It took decades until these plants came to be considered again as compounds of therapeutic value and medical use, though its uses are highly restricted.

The cannabis plant originated in Central Asia, but today it is grown worldwide and considered to be one of the most popular plants. In the United States, it's a controlled substance by government agencies and is classified as a Schedule I agent; this implies that it's a drug with increased potential for abuse hence there is a caution in the sale and use of the drug.

Numerous diseases and infections which include; **anorexia, emesis, pain, anxieties, inflammation, multiple sclerosis, neurodegenerative disorders, Asthma, epilepsy, glaucoma, Osteoporosis, schizophrenia, cardiovascular disorders, cancer, obesity, skin treatment**, and **metabolic syndrome**-related disorders are known to be treated or have the potential to be treated with cannabis oils and other cannabinoid compounds.

Though research and studies into cannabis oil are limited due to strict government guidelines and limitations in accessing it, a growing number of pediatric patients are also seeking symptom relief with cannabis or cannabinoid treatment, and it has been a quick solution to other problems. This book is a product of deep research into the medicinal importance and other benefits of cannabis oil. It is enriched with so many health issues that cannabis oil has been found to cure.

Copyright 2018 by Martin Pals - All rights reserved.

This document is geared towards providing exact and reliable information in regards to the topic and issue covered. The publication is sold with the idea that the publisher is not required to render accounting, officially permitted, or otherwise, qualified services. If advice is necessary, legal or professional, a practiced individual in the profession should be ordered.

- From a Declaration of Principles which was accepted and approved equally by a Committee of the American Bar Association and a Committee of Publishers and Associations.

In no way is it legal to reproduce, duplicate, or transmit any part of this document in either electronic means or in printed format. Recording of this publication is strictly prohibited and any storage of this document is not allowed unless with written permission from the publisher. All rights reserved.

The information provided herein is stated to be truthful and consistent, in that any liability, in terms of inattention or otherwise, by any usage or abuse of any policies, processes, or directions contained within is the solitary and utter responsibility of the recipient reader. Under no circumstances will any legal responsibility or blame be held against the publisher for any reparation, damages, or monetary loss due to the information herein, either directly or indirectly.

Respective authors own all copyrights not held by the publisher.

The information herein is offered for informational purposes solely, and is universal as so. The presentation of the information is without contract or any type of guarantee assurance.

The trademarks that are used are without any consent, and the publication of the trademark is without permission or backing by the trademark owner. All trademarks and brands within this book are for clarifying purposes only and are the owned by the owners themselves, not affiliated with this document.

Components of Cannabis Oil

Cannabinoids, which are components of cannabis oil, are a group of a 21-carbon compound containing terpene-phenolic compounds that are produced expressly by cannabis species. These compounds may be referred to as phytocannabinoids.

Although delta-9-tetrahydrocannabinol (the THC) is the primary psychoactive ingredient of the cannabinoids, there are other known compounds with active biologic activity; these compounds include cannabinol, cannabidiol, cannabichromene, cannabigerol, tetrahydrocannabivarin, and popular delta-8-THC.

Cannabidiol is known to have significant pain, stress-relieving, and anti-inflammatory activity even in the absence of the psychoactive effect of delta-9-THC.

How to Obtain and Use Cannabis

Individuals who use cannabis oil as a means of treating different health conditions ingest it into their body with an oral syringe or by adding it to a fluid that masks its potency. The dose measurement and frequency are mainly based on the health condition being treated and the patient's cannabis tolerance level; this level can be ascertained through a doctor or health expert. Most patients often start with a small amount and then increase the treatment doses over a long period depending on their cannabis tolerance level. You need to know your level of tolerance to avoid abusing this drug.

It's difficult if not impossible to buy cannabis oil online or at a local pharmaceutical store, the reason is not far-fetched as there are huge regulations on the sales of the oil. Some states provide individuals with cannabis strictly for medical conditions, and this may require a medical note or proof of injury and illness from a hospital to qualify to access this drug. Also, to access it, you can also join a collective health group, which is a group of patients who grow and share medical cannabis with a legal right to do so. If you are to use cannabis oil, make sure it's purchased from a reputable company that has the legal right to sell pure and lab-tested oils to people.

Fake cannabis oils online

There are many fake cannabis oils online, and most of them are imported and sold to patients who are in dire need of this oil. This is why it is good to read books and ask questions before paying for any cannabis oil.

Some of the cannabis which is seen online is adulterated and wrongly produced and should not be used in treating any health problem. Medical experts recommend that you go through the legal and safe means of obtaining cannabis oil to ensure its health benefits and avoid any possible side effects.

As a word of caution, please do not use cannabis oil, or any cannabis product, or any cannabidiol drug if you are pregnant or could become pregnant within a short time!

There is some available evidence which suggests that women who use cannabis oil or products during the time of conception or while pregnant may increase the risk of their child being born with possible birth defects or at a very low weight, also breastfeeding mothers are advised not to use this drug.

Cannabis Oil

Cannabis is a very powerful medicinal herb with a very long history of curing many health problems and skin infections. According to medical history accrued over the years, cannabis has been cultivated in various regions of the world for millennia, and its cultivation has grown with time as a result of its frequent demand and medical purpose.

Cannabis, which is also known as **marijuana**, refers to the liquids or oil derived from the **Cannabis Sativa plant**, which is typically cultivated for their potent trichomes and other important usages. These seemingly sticky glands contain high amounts of a substance which is referred to as THC or tetrahydrocannabinol, a substance known for its psychotropic abilities and cancer curing capacity.

Cannabis oil is found to be a strong and sticky resinous substance that is derived from the cannabis plant and which has found to be of great importance in the medical world. This oil has become very popular and infamous in recent years due to the movement for legalized marijuana in some countries as opposed to the laws imposed on its transportation from different parts of the world. Found to possess CBD and THC, there are a good number of health benefits that users of cannabis oil derive from it.

It is deduced from the resin of the cannabis flowers. Due to the increasing number of health issues that cannabis oil has been found to solve, it is becoming a clarion call for all to take advantage of the numerous uses of this herb. This book is written so that the reader will gain useful insights on how to use cannabis oil in solving those problems that the use of chemical drugs has been unable to solve.

Cannabis is being transported to different countries and has found usefulness, though largely misused. It has different names, according to drugs.com. Cannabis is also known as Ganja, Grass, Hashish, Hemp, Indian hemp, marijuana, Pot, reefer, weed, and lots of different names given to it in various countries of the world.

Extracting the Cannabis Oil

To extract cannabis oil from the Sativa plant, a solvent extraction process is used during this process, which returns roughly 3-5 grams of oil per ounce of flower product that is used during the extraction. You can also use grain alcohol or isopropyl alcohol as a solvent during the extraction process, and you will then strain the result of the mixture, which will leave cannabis oil as the residue.

This process is a rather involved and lengthy process that requires the use of some equipment to achieve, and in countries where cannabis is legal, there are many places to access high-quality cannabis oil that has already been extracted. It is my prediction that though the cannabis leaf is widely misused, in the long term this oil will be a breakthrough in the medical world as enough research is currently ongoing on the usefulness of this oil. This oil is also seen to be a very good skin nourishing oil, and one is forced to ask why this important oil with such medical uses is so strictly limited and restricted.

The importance of Cannabis Oil

The medical importance of this oil cannot be over-emphasized. Cannabis oil has a wide range of effects on human health, and it has been linked to a diverse number of health challenges and issues, ranging from migraines and stress to lack of appetite and low sex drive in humans.

Cannabis oil has even been connected to reducing the risk of certain cancers even more than chemical drugs can do, as well as reduce body pains. It is also known to help in strengthening the heart and helping people get a good night's sleep after a very stressful day or after strenuous activities.

There are some ways to use cannabis oil in solving many health problems, depending on what you want relief from; it can be useful in treating virtually any issues as well as in treating some known skin infections.

10 Health treatments using Cannabis Oil

Medical Research into cannabis essential oil is highly regulated, and science is still in the early stages of its development and uses of the oil. It is the hope of science that in the nearest future, as technology is evolving in the medical direction that more research will be conducted and that the regulatory bodies restricting the use of cannabis oil will become more welcoming to its potential to treat people safely without any side effects or complications.

Therefore let's look at the health benefits of using cannabis oil.

1. Stress and Anxiety

Stress, anxiety, and other related emotional disorders are an increasing modern concern that is fast spreading and has a strong base in the United States. The medical world is continuously looking at numerous potential and natural alternatives in resolving emotional disorders. There have been many highly ineffective and dangerous prescriptions used to treat these disorders, and there is a need for an alternative. On average, **almost 6 in every 10 Americans** suffer from stress and anxiety on a daily basis, while they have traditionally relied on drugs to get over this stress, the high increase of this disorder is a sure proof that a better alternative is needed in solving this problem.

Cannabis oil is, therefore, worth exploring and studying further as it can relax the troubled mind and stimulate the release of pleasure hormones in the bodies of those that use it. This combination of effects can lead to speedy stress reduction and provide a way for feelings of calmness and general well being of the entire body. As has been pointed out in the sections above, cannabis oil can help in getting a sound night's sleep/rest which is known to reduce anxiety and stress.

Cannabinoids which are found in the oil are responsible for creating a positive emotional response in the body's nervous system as it helps to relax the entire system and prepare the body for work later on. Several recent studies have demonstrated the potential value of cannabis oil in stress relief as well as solving other related issues like insomnia.

One recent study that reveals this is an Israeli study which was published in 2013, which demonstrated that treating the body with cannabinoids following some form of traumatic experience might help to reduce and control the emotional responses to that traumatic event and prevent stress-related responses gotten as a result of a traumatic experience.

Researchers also discovered that cannabinoids were effective in reducing stress receptors in the body's hippocampus, which is the area of the brain responsible for emotional response and control of trauma.

Also, cannabis treatments were found to be very effective in reducing anxiety and restlessness in military veterans who are suffering from PTSD. Whether cannabis oil is inhaled or orally administered, it leads to a wide range of positive nervous system effects that include an increased feeling of body pleasure and calmness. While there is a need for further research on how cannabis oil can help in stress relief, the research conducted so far as well as a large body of anecdotal evidence found has been very promising for the future use of cannabis oil to treat anxiety, stress, and sleeping disorders. The natural compounds found in cannabis oil like THC, which gives the cannabis a drug classification, are very good for the release of the pleasure homes as has been discussed above.

Also for people who suffer from insomnia and constant anxiety during the nighttime hours or those who always struggle to get a sound, restful night of undisturbed sleep, you need to worry no more as cannabis oil works like a charm in getting you to easily fall asleep and sustaining you throughout the whole night's sleep. By relaxing your body, mind, and by inducing a lower energy level in your body, it will be easier to get your heartbeat rate down and clear your head to prepare you for a long night of peaceful slumber without any of the body aches or anxiety that you might have experienced before.

2. Appetite and Obesity

Cannabis has a well-known history of its ability to increase an individual's appetite for food. It is also possible that it has potential to be a good supplement for people who need to increase their weight as a result of a sickness that made them lose a lot of weight or because of an eating disorder like anorexia nervosa that can induce a weight loss in the body.

Cannabis oil can serve as a stimulant to the body's digestive system and induce hunger in those lacking the appetite to eat. While cannabis oil can induce taste for food by helping release hormones responsible for hunger, it is important that some certain hormones responsible for hunger suppression can also be stimulated by cannabinoids which are found in cannabis oil.

In summary, depending on which hormone gets stimulated in the long run, cannabis oil might also be very effective in reducing appetite and controlling obesity in the body of those its users. To effectively control obesity, it is important to manipulate the cannabinoids in cannabis oil to stimulate the appropriate hormones for any purpose in which it is used to achieve.

Cannabis oil may be very much effective in treating both obesity and eating disorders like anorexia simultaneously in the nearest future.

Therefore those who wish to reduce weight can take refuge in cannabis oil to achieve a quick result. If you have been looking for an appetite booster, look no more.

3. Asthma

Asthma is a general respiratory disease that affects up to 300 million people around the world. Asthma is responsible for numerous deaths every year, and the search for a natural and effective treatment to curtail the growth and propagation of this ailment has been ongoing for many years and will remain at the forefront of research in the medical world.

So the million-dollar question is how cannabis oil can help in the treatment of Asthma.

Cannabis has been traditionally used to treat asthma for many years in Chinese and Indian medicine. With such capabilities, cannabis oil may be an effective natural treatment for asthmatic patients because of its natural anti-inflammatory ability and its ability to dilate the bronchial tubes, which are a pathway for in the inflow of oxygen into the respiratory system.

It should be known that during the early 1970s there were several research studies which investigated the bronchodilatory effects of cannabis for people suffering from asthma and most of this research was positive—hence, it can be said to be a good drug for treating Asthma. While there is little available evidence regarding the use of cannabis oil for asthmatics it has been found to improve the symptoms of Asthma and hence could be used in its treatment and cure. Also, early reports have revealed the presence of an active ingredient in cannabis essential oil that can prevent the effects of Asthma.

4. Heart Health

As cannabis oil continues to be a good alternative for the treatment of many physical problems, the heart is not left out. This is because cannabis oil contains active antioxidant properties that have proven to be very beneficial for the total wellbeing and functioning of the heart. Animal studies conducted to this effect have demonstrated that treatment with cannabis oil can prevent numerous cardiovascular diseases most of which include: atherosclerosis, heart attacks, catarrh, and strokes.

This animal study finds application to human heart conditions; this is because the cannabinoids could cause the blood vessels to relax further and dilate creating the pathway to improved blood and air circulation and also reduced blood pressure within the heart. This study is a breakthrough, and other forthcoming studies will further prove that cannabis oil has major implications for the health of the heart.

This study also reveals that those who regularly consume cannabis oil have a reduced chance of having a stroke. The increasing number of stroke is drawing a global concern, so anything that can prevent it especially important to know.

5. Pain Relief

One of the popular historical applications of the cannabis plant oil has been to ease pains and inflammation in the body.

There is evidence that cannabis oil has been used for thousands of years to resolve these purposes. Also, there is corresponding modern evidence that shows cannabis and cannabis oil is effective in relieving body pain and inflammation by inhibiting the neural transmission in the body's pain pathways such that the neural transmission does not get to go deep into the body. The cannabis oil has the potential to cure chronic pain as well as inflammation, which is why many cancer patients all over the world choose to take it while undergoing chemotherapy and medical experts have highly recommended it.

Many people often take cannabis oil to deal with severe rheumatism and arthritis as well as other chronic pains found in the body especially among the older ones. Other recent research has demonstrated that it can be used to alleviate neuropathic pain in most patients. It is considered to be very safe when taken in appropriate prescriptions, and studies have found that it is largely well tolerated, unlike the leaf which is widely misused by many.

6. Cancer

There has been a considerable amount of excitement in the medical world regarding the ability of cannabis oil to cure cancer. This great news often makes headlines or published in most medical journals. Unfortunately, these headlines are often overly optimistic and can be misleading for both patients and their families who do not truly understand the truth of what cannabis oil can do and the things it cannot do to cancer patients.

First of all, it should be clearly stated out that the large majority of scientific research into the effects of cannabis oil in treating cancer had been conducted either on animals or in the laboratory. The implication is that we need to exercise a degree of caution in extrapolating the results to human subjects; however, the fact that the results gotten so far reveals it can cure cancer in a human. If any drug for treating the cancerous cells is discovered, it is first tried with animals to check the effect before using it on humans. This is achieved by injecting cancerous cells in the body of the animal, which in most cases a rat is used since it is a mammal. Then the cancer cells are allowed to get hold of the animal before the potential treatment is injected and watched to observe the effect of it in treating the disease.

In light of this testimony, scientists have been able to discover that many different cannabinoids in the cannabis plant have a range of positive effects under laboratory conditions in treating cancer.

These positive effects include:

- Triggering the immediate death of the cancer cells, this process is commonly known as apoptosis.

- Preventing and reducing the division of cancerous cells.

- Preventing new blood vessels from becoming tumors which lead to the formation of cancer in the body of the victim.

- Reducing the risk and rate of cancerous cells from spreading throughout the body and attacking the healthy neighboring tissue.

It should be known that up to now the most positive effects results have been seen when using a combination of purified THC in combination with cannabidiol. This is a cannabinoid that counteracts the psychoactive effect of THC, and a more positive result is observed on a daily basis.

Other medical research has revealed that cannabis oil is highly effective when used in combination with other chemotherapy medications in treating cancer. Although there is no hard and fast evidence that cannabis oil is a miracle cure-all for cancer treatment, the early signs are very glaring, and further research into it will soon help us find the answers that the world is earnestly waiting for.

As has been pointed out in this paragraph, the com-bination of cannabis oil and other chemotherapy has proven to be useful in treating cancer. This is one of the recent improvements in the medical world as so many people suffer from cancer and any treatment of this is a quantum leap.

Another treatment of cancer, which is gaining more attention in the health industry, is the use of nano-technology, though for now, it is still the product of laboratory investigation. Treating with cannabis oil remains the safest for now since it has no side effect and it has proven to be successful.

When treating cancer, the suggestion is always to take three doses of cannabis oil each day, and subsequently, increase the amount of the dose until 1 gram per day is consumed on daily. A full treatment of cancer is believed to take 90 days if the patient follows the prescriptions. It should be known that the sale of cannabis oil is still illegal in many countries though it can be gotten in the United States. The process of getting it has been explained above. Though due to the significant amount of research being done on its medical applications and usage, and some reputable sources and agencies have put out guides for the access and use of cannabis oil for the treatment of the cancer disease. Hence this oil can be sought with permission and may not be allowed to be imported from other countries, especially from countries where its use is illegal. Thus, when searching online for this oil, you must be very observant to avoid being scammed by fake online dealers.

7. Skin Protection

Cannabis oil can be used topically to maintain healthy and glowing skin. When applied topically on the skin, cannabis oil can help stimulate the shedding of older and dead skin cells, exfoliation of the skin, and promote the growth of new skin cells to replace the older ones. Applying cannabis oil, as well as aloe after-sun gel, witch hazel, tea tree oil or other aloe-based lotion after shaving can help the skin feel cool, relaxed, comfortable, and may help keep it smooth later. You may also try using radiant skin silk body lotion or other lotion recommended by a dermatologist, which has calming calendula, chamomile, and sunflower oil on your skin as it will help retain your skin color. But the cannabis is a good treatment for the skin even for razor bumps.

Cannabinoids can aid to enhance the production of lipids, which help fight chronic skin conditions including razor bumps, acne, and psoriasis. There is a possibility that cannabis oil can help prevent the signs of aging like wrinkles, skin spots, blemishes. And other body aging signs on the body because it is high in natural antioxidants that help fight against cellular damage caused by free radicals and help to nourish the skin to be smooth and ever glowing. One of the most powerful uses of cannabis is in the protection of the skin. To achieve this, cannabis oil can be consumed or applied externally on the skin as it has been most effective. By reducing the effect and amount of stress that we feel inside the body, cannabis oil can also be very helpful in preventing skin diseases that tend to break out during times of anxiety and stress like eczema or rosacea.

This is the reason while the global demand for cannabis oil is growing astronomically because of the need to maintain the skin color and beauty.

8. Eye Health

There is available evidence which demonstrates the ability and usefulness of cannabis oil to treat some eye conditions like glaucoma and macular degeneration, which is common among many people. Glaucoma is a serious optic nerve disease of the eye that might lead to loss of proper vision and even total blindness when not properly managed or treated.

Glaucoma is caused by the accumulation of fluid within the eye, which results in too much pressure on the retina, lens, and optic nerve of the eyes. While numerous factors may contribute to nerve damage in many people suffering from glaucoma, it is completely related and linked to intraocular pressure or IOP.

The American Glaucoma Society has confirmed the place of cannabis oil in treating this eye problem. The society reveals that cannabis oil can reduce the level of IOP in both those suffering from glaucoma and the potential glaucoma patients. Unfortunately, its effects in solving the IOP level on the eyes are temporary, and patients would need to use cannabis oil only for few hours to shore up the effects as we expect more research on its ability to completely cure the eye problem.

9. For Treating Seizures

Though there has been some controversy over this, there is still some evidence emanating from small-scale studies carried out using cannabis oil. This anecdotal report suggests that the cannabidiol content of cannabis oil can be very useful in preventing seizures and could be used as a novel treatment for epilepsy in humans.

Though the truth is that there is not enough evidence to back up its use in treating seizures and the limited evidence that is available so far has proven contradictory among some scientists. Among the seizure patients who were treated with cannabis oil, it should be noted that of none of them experienced any adverse side effects as a result of the treatment and that more studies in future may prove to be very useful in treating this problem.

10. Other Potential Benefits of the Cannabis oil

Headaches and Migraines:

It has been proven that cannabis oil is an effective tool in the treatment of migraines and headache. When the oil is topically applied at the temples or the spot of intensity for a migraine or a headache, it is found to be an effective way to get relief. As a result of this, many people obtain prescriptions for cannabis and cannabis oil due to its potent defense against crippling headaches and other body pain. Hence it is very useful for getting quick relief when having a headache.

The United States' laws on the Cannabis Oil

The use and sale of cannabis and cannabis oil for medicinal purposes are now legalized in 25 states in the United States though you shouldn't expect to be able to walk into a shop and buy it as you may not see it sold in public stores or pharmacists. To have access to this product, you may require a medical certificate and a proof of illness to acquire cannabis oil from the state, but you can obtain this proof easily, and you will be given access to it.

To have quick access to this product, you may have to join a collective group, i.e., a group of patients that share and sometimes grow medicinal cannabis due to their health problems. This method remains the fastest means of getting access to cannabis oil. Or you can further contact me on how to go about getting this in oil.

You need to be aware that there are numerous scams and fake dealers online promising to sell medicinal cannabis to you. These persons only aim at deceiving you and getting away with your money. Hence it is very important that you do your research and find a well-known dealer well before you go ahead with your purchase. Experts' advise that you purchase only oil produced by a reputable company who test the product in a lab, so you don't have complications or don't find yourself deceived into using fake cannabis in treating your problems.

The Difference between the Cannabis oil and Hemp oil

Often, many people confuse the two without having proper knowledge of what the difference between the two herbs. It is pertinent to know that both cannabis and hemp oil are derived from the same species, the "Cannabis sativa." Unlike cannabis oil, hemp oil is quite different due to its production. Therefore, hemp is a high growing species of the plant Sativa, which is commonly produced for industrial purposes like topical ointments, fiber, paper, and other industrial purposes.

Unlike cannabis oil, hemp oil has only trace amounts of THC (in little quantity) and hence is not considered to have the same medicinal value as that of cannabis oil. It is also important to know that both hemp oil and cannabis oil also contain the cannabidiol or CBD, which contain medicinal properties, notwithstanding, cannabis oil is of good medicinal value as compared to hemp oil.

However, it is found that there is far less of this compound (THC) contained in hemp than cannabis oil, hence the superiority of cannabis oil over hemp in solving medical issues. According to results of the recent study, cannabis oil is actually around 100 times more potent than hemp oil; this implies that the dose of hemp oil necessary to have an equivalent medicinal effect would be extremely high and less cost effective. This research further speaks of the need for the use of cannabis oil over hemp for a quick result in any health-related issue.

Word of Caution

Although this list clearly outlines that cannabis oil can be an effective remedy for treating many common health conditions, it should be remembered that it is still a potent chemical substance extracted from a plant with high psychotropic substances and hence caution should be taken. Therefore, users should always be very careful in the way and manner cannabis oil is used, this includes the conditions under which the oil is taken. It is advisable that you speak to a professional about combining the oil and present medications before adding any new elements to your health regimen to avoid any complications that may result from the chemical reactions. Also, the use of cannabis oil is restricted/banned by many countries, so it is necessary that you consult local health specialists before you use cannabis oil.

Conclusion

Cannabis is a plant genus which is of three different species: Indica, Sativa, and Ruderalis, and it's been used for both health and medicinal purposes for thousands of years and is still a current trend in the medical world. Cannabis oil has been used in the treatment of many diseases without any side effects or complications. I have to accept the fact that a mild addiction to cannabis is possible, but medical researchers agree that the therapeutic effects of cannabinoids are considerable and should not be ignored. In particular, uses for cannabis oil cannot be stopped or neglected since it has numerous advantages than disadvantages. There is also a method of checking an individual's cannabis tolerance level which makes the use of the oil to be moderated and not be abused.

Smoking marijuana leaf is well known to increase appetite in a person, but the cannabis essential oil can also help to stimulate your digestive system and induce hunger. This ability of cannabis oil is useful for people who are trying to gain weight, especially after an illness or injury which led to the loss of body weight. Cannabis leaf and cannabis oil have also been linked to the prevention of macular degeneration and the treatment of glaucoma especially among the aged persons in the society. As one grows older, cannabis oil is useful in ensuring the total wellbeing of the body. It can keep an individual safe from diseases which is associated with old age. Although research is still ongoing, cannabis oil is considered an option in the treatment and prevention of cancer as the available research has suggested. Using cannabis oil in cancer prevention or treatment may help reduce tumor size and alleviate possible weakness, pain, nausea, and a lack of appetite in a cancer patient. Cannabis oil may improve the health of cancer patients by triggering cancer cell death and cutting off the pathway of the blood supply to the tumor. Other case reports into the cancer treatment have found that cannabis oil is a non-toxic chemotherapy alternative that has the ability to increase vitality in patients with acute lymphoblastic leukemia.

Aside its usefulness in treating to diseases, Cannabinoids found in cannabis produce lipids, which can help treat dry skin, dandruff or acne, and help to improve the skin's appearance. The oil is also seen to fight any free-radical damage on the skin and reduce the stress linked with eczema, rosacea, and acne. In fact, cannabis oil is generally used for the total skin treatment; there are also cannabis oil benefits for the hair. Veterinary studies on animals have revealed that cannabis may prevent heart conditions such as heart attacks, atherosclerosis, stroke, hypertension, and coronary heart disease, which is also applicable to the human. Post-traumatic stress disorder (PTSD) is a common psychiatric condition that results from life-threatening experiences such as military wars or combats, serious accidents, or natural disasters, and emotional trauma. From the above, it is very visible to the blind and audible to the deaf that cannabis oil is very important if anyone must live a healthy life.

CANNABIS COOKBOOK

> Marijuana-infused food is booming!
>
> This cannabis cookbook includes meals for every moment and more useful information about cannabis.

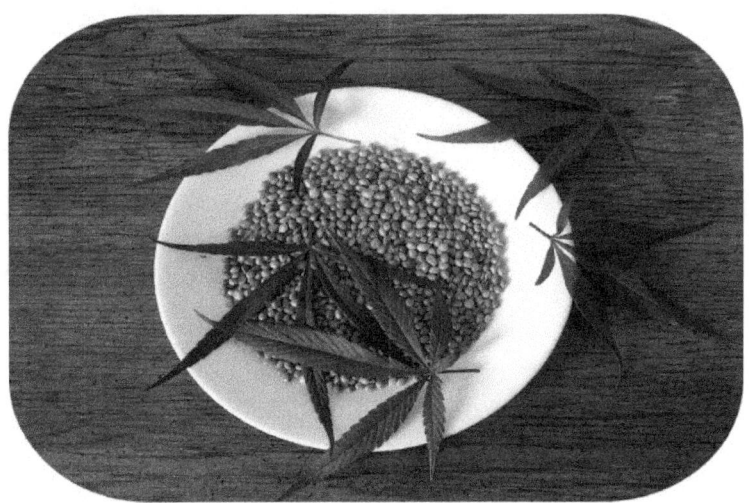

Martin Pals

Introduction

I want to thank you and congratulate you for getting this Cannabis Cookbook.

This book contains recipes with cannabis as a central ingredient and additional information on cannabis.

In this book, I will teach you to create great tasting food, with an extra element: the effect of the ingredient marijuana.

Cannabis is edible and is popular around the world. This herb is not eaten in a regular sort of way but eaten recreationally.

The herb has some potential effects on the human body when taken in measured quantity. There is an increase in energy in a person who takes it. It goes by several names like weed, pot, marijuana.

Cannabis is taken in small amounts and only a pinch of powdered cannabis is sufficient to bring about the effects.

The most common recipes that use cannabis are cookies and brownies. The recipes are the same as usual except that there is a small amount of pot added. No one likes the taste of cannabis or wants to taste the herb on their tongue, so only add it in small amounts.

Most of these simple recipes use canna-butter or canna-oil. Cannabis contains THC which is responsible for humans getting high from consuming it. If eaten straight, the weed tastes disgusting and the digestive system will not be able to absorb the THC. Hence, weed has to be manipulated in some way for the THC to work.

It is important to know the properties of cannabis. THC is fat soluble. Cook it in fat or oil and not water. The most common thing to do with it is to prepare canna-butter or canna-oil that you can use for cooking.

Some recipes use butter and others use oil. The most commonly used oils are coconut and olive. Canola is also used.

Thanks again for downloading this book, I hope you enjoy it and enjoy your meals!

© Copyright 2017 by Martin Pals - All rights reserved.

This document is geared towards providing exact and reliable information in regard to the topic and issue covered. The publication is sold with the idea that the publisher is not required to render accounting, officially permitted, or otherwise, qualified services. If advice is necessary, legal or professional, a practiced individual in the profession should be consulted.

- From a Declaration of Principles which was accepted and approved equally by a Committee of the American Bar Association and a Committee of Publishers and Associations.

In no way is it legal to reproduce, duplicate, or transmit any part of this document in either electronic means or in printed format. Recording of this publication is strictly prohibited and any storage of this document is not allowed unless with written permission from the publisher. All rights reserved.

The information provided herein is stated to be truthful and consistent, in that any liability, in terms of inattention or otherwise, by any usage or abuse of any policies, processes, or directions contained within is the solitary and utter responsibility of the reader. Under no circumstances will any legal responsibility or blame be held against the publisher for any reparation, damages, or monetary loss due to the information herein, either directly or indirectly.

Respective authors own all copyrights not held by the publisher.

The information herein is offered solely for informational purposes, and is universal as so. The presentation of the information is without contract or any type of guarantee assurance.

The trademarks that are used are without any consent, and the publication of the trademark is without permission or backing by the trademark owner. All trademarks and brands within this book are for clarifying purposes only and are the owned by the owners themselves, not affiliated with this document.

Contents

Introduction ....

Understand What Cannabis Is ....

    An Understanding of Cannabis 7

    Who Uses Cannabis? 8

    Why Cannabis is Widely Used by People? 9

    Short-Term Effects of Cannabis 9

    Long-Term Effects of Cannabis 9

What happens while you smoke or eat cannabis? ....

Health benefits of Cannabis ....

The Difference Between Cannabis and Other Psychoactive Drugs ....

    Cannabis as Psychoactive Drugs 15

    Other Psychoactive Drugs 16

Remedies for a cannabis overdose ....

Basics Cannabis ingredients ....

    Steps to make Canna-butter 20

    How to make Canna-oil? 23

Drinks ....

    Cannabis Milkshake 25

    Have a Drink with Cannabis Hot Chocolate 27

Meals ....

    How to Make Crispy Cannabis Tacos 30

It's Time to Try Delicious Cannaburger Recipe 33

Delectable Cannabis Spaghetti Sauce Recipe 36

Make Skirt Steak Salad with Cannabis ....

Desserts / Snacks ....

Recipe for Cananbis Chocolate Chip Cookies 42

How to Make Mouth-Watering Cannabis Dark Chocolate Covered Blueberry Clusters 45

Classic Special Brownies' Recipe 48

Nutella high biscuits 51

Give a treat to your taste buds with Frozen Trifle Dessert infused with marijuana 53

Cannabis-infused candy recipes that are easy to make 56

Canna Gummy 56

Canna Rangers 56

Cannaghee –based jalebis 57

Coconut cannabis covered raisins. 57

Conclusion ....

Check Out My Other Books ....

Understand What Cannabis Is

Derived from the sativa of cannabis plant, cannabis usually grows in many temperate and tropical areas in the world. One great thing about this plant is that it can be grown in any climate and, with the help of indoor hydroponic technology, it has been increasingly cultivated in many places.

The active ingredient found in cannabis is delta-9 tetrahydro-cannabinol, popularly known as THC. Because of this, the plant gives the 'high'. Due to its potency, THC can produce a wide range of products.

An Understanding of Cannabis

Cannabis is basically used in three different forms;

- Marijuana
- Hashish
- Hash oil

Derived from the dried flowers and leaves of the cannabis plant, marijuana is made. Among all the cannabis products, marijuana is the least potent. It is usually used for smoking and into different edible products such as cookies and brownies.

Another form of cannabis —hashish is derived from the resin or a secreted gum of this plant. This resin is dried and then pressed into tiny blocks and smoked. Hashish is also used in foods. The most potent cannabis product is hash oil or cannabis oil. This thick oil is derived from hashish and it is also smoked.

> **Different Names of Cannabis**
>
> Cannabis is called many different names such as marijuana, dope, pot, weed, hooch, Mary Jane, joints, grass, cones, smoke, brew, hydro, green, mull and so on.

Who Uses Cannabis?

Throughout the United States, cannabis is considered as the most widely used illegal drug. A survey conducted by the National Survey on Drug Use and Health revealed that 7.3% of Americans aged 12 years or above have taken marijuana, while the average age for the first-time user is 17.9 years.

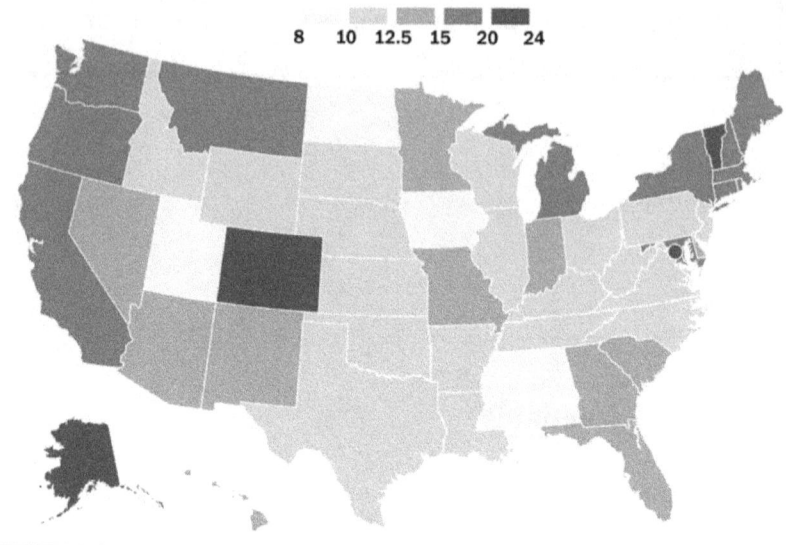

Although the use of marijuana among the youth has remained relatively stable in the last several years, the youth perception of the harmful effects of marijuana has been gradually reducing which means a smaller number of adolescents consider the effects of this drug harmful. At present, marijuana comes next to alcohol in respect of most-commonly used substances.

Why Cannabis is Widely Used by People?

Cannabis can produce a sense of mild euphoria and relaxation and therefore, many people take it to get such experience as they refer to it as a 'high'. Cannabis can bring changes in the user's mood and impact their thoughts and perceptions of the environment. In this connection, cannabis is also used for beneficial purposes to overcome depression in medical science.

It is also true that cannabis has many helpful benefits on human life and therefore, cannabis is used in medical science for different kinds of treatments ranging from cancer to diabetes and depression.

Short-Term Effects of Cannabis

The short-term effects of taking cannabis include:

- Drowsiness
- Feeling of well-being
- Talkativeness
- Loss of co-ordination
- Increased appetite and decreased nausea
- Bloodshot eyes

Long-Term Effects of Cannabis

Limited research has been conducted to find out the long-term effects of cannabis.

From the available evidence, effects like increased risk of respiratory diseases related to smoking, decreased motivation in work, study and other fields and reduced memory and learning capacities have been observed as its adverse effect.

What happens while you smoke or eat cannabis?

Even if you have not consumed or smoked cannabis in your life, you can experience similar kinds of things. It is possible to come across a giggling attitude following consumption of the herb. Sudden desire may erupt in your mind. Old memories may come back as you discuss subjects from school days. Some overt symptoms can also be noticed at the time. Diverse kinds of effects can be seen throughout the body following a cannabis smoking episode. Hidden processes within the body can be seen at the time.

The function of smoking and eating cannabis is vague. Infusion of THC can be noticed through the blood stream and interaction with the brain can be noticed at the time. The orbito-frontal cortex and tetrahydrocannabinol is affected mostly on occasion. The concept is complicated; therefore, the process may not be easy to understand at all.

Knowledge of a layman may not be effective. Overt symptoms are generally discussed such as red eyes. However, you know what goes inside your body too. Lots of research has been done to achieve a solution. Research may go on in the future also. The following things may be observed with smoking or eating cannabis.

Flooding the Brain with Dopamine

Due to neurotransmitter dopamine, a high is experienced with Dopamine. The reward system of the brain is also associated with the situation. It is possible to observe action through cannabinoid receptors. Huge amounts of dopamine can be released which may stimulate the THC and a euphoric feeling can be enjoyed.

Drying up of Body Fluid

Most people consider cannabis as a type of mood killer. Mucus membrane can dry up with excessive use of the herb. Expansion of blood vessels can occur and fluids can dry up in some other parts of the body too.

Drop in Blood Pressure

Dilation of blood vessels can be noticed as cannabis is infused with the blood. It may lead to a drop in blood pressure. This effect can be noticed most prominently through the eyes which may become red. As a result, the pupil must be dilated.

Sense becomes intense

Cannabis consumption or smoking heightens senses. Therefore, you may be able to get a smell or a taste more markedly. Side effects like pupil dilation may be noticed at the time too. Other senses may be developed too.

Increased Heart Rate

Heart rate may be enhanced due to use of cannabis. The effect of the herb can be noticed for almost three hours. The process may not cause any harm at all, however, increase in the rate of heart attack can be noticed. Issues may occur with decrease in the blood pressure level.

Fooling the feeding system of the brain

Incorrect messages regarding appetite may be sent to the brain. Previously, it has been thought that cannabis enhances your appetite. However, a 2015 study has revealed that cannabis signals the body to start the process of eating.

Health benefits of Cannabis

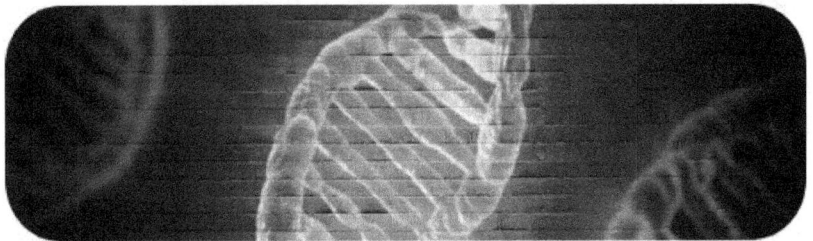

Not everyone may believe that cannabis is a magical herb. In this article, the health benefits of cannabis are discussed to inform you what can be done with cannabis. From health to economy can benefit from this herb. By developing a positive relationship with this plant, you may able to enjoy its therapeutic benefits.

Lose Weight

Through research, it has been found that cannabis helps to reduce your weight easily. Slimming of average nature may be noticed at the time. Insulin production can be regulated perfectly with daily use of this herb. Caloric intake can be managed also.

Prevention and regulation of Diabetes

Due to regulation of body weight, diabetes can be prevented in the same manner too. Cannabis can be considered as a breakthrough for diabetics. Therefore, the drug can be used quite naturally for your health.

Fighting Cancer

One of the biggest advantages of cannabis can be the prevention of cancer. Scientist as well as the federal government have released evidence that cannabis can deal with specific kinds of cancer. Therefore, it can be utilized quite substantially.

Avoiding Depression

Most people in the world suffer from depression at some stage in life. It has often been considered as a medical condition in the United States of America. Treatment of depression may be possible through use of cannabis. Through cannabis, it may be possible to retain the normal function of the endocannabinoid. In this way, mood stabilization is possible. In addition, you may be able to come out of depression too with current research occurring right now. Therefore, more concrete results will be found in the future.

Treatment of Autism

Like several other disorders, autism can also be treated with the assistance of cannabis. Scientists have been looking in to matter seriously. However, parents are also using this drug to deal with the mood swings in the autistic children. Behavior can be stabilized in due course.

Substitute for alcohol and drugs

Harmful results can be noticed with the use of cannabis if it is not handled with care. However, it may not produce similar kinds of destructive result as alcohol. If cannabis has been made widely available, then it may become a suitable alternative to alcohol and drugs. Lives can be saved as a result.

Regulating seizures

Seizures can be controlled with the use of medical cannabis. These findings have been seen from the world of medical science. Huge amounts of promise have been showcased by cannabis for Epilepsy.

Broken bones can be healed much faster

Do you think that cannabis can heal bones? Chemical reaction between cannabis and collagen can mend the bones perfectly. It can be considered one of the remarkable finds about this herb.

Curing ADHD

If you have trouble concentrating, then you may be suffering from ADHD or ADD. Cannabis can be utilized for the treatment of this condition. The safety and effectiveness of the cannabis cannot be doubted.

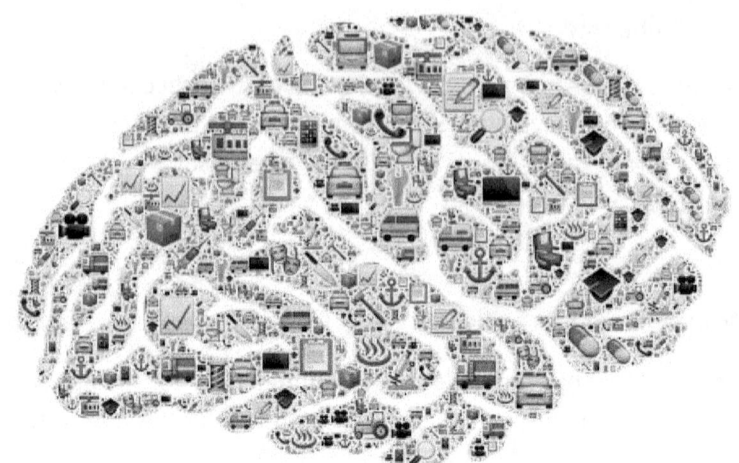

The Difference Between Cannabis and Other Psychoactive Drugs

Psychoactive drugs have the potency to affect the central nervous system and alter the consciousness, thoughts and moods of the users. Different types of psychoactive drugs include cannabis, alcohol, cocaine, heroin, ecstasy and amphetamines. Psychoactive drugs can be categorized into different groups:

- **Depressants:** Certain psychoactive drugs can reduce alertness by slowing down the activities operated by the central nervous system. Examples of such depressants are alcohol, heroin and analgesics.

- **Stimulants**: Some psychoactive drugs can increase the state of arousal in the body by increasing the brain's activity. Examples are tobacco, caffeine and amphetamines.

- **Hallucinogens**: Drugs such as LSD and 'magic mushrooms' can alter perception and create hallucination.

- **Other Psychoactive Drugs**: Apart from these three categories, some drugs belong to the 'other' category since they have more than one of these categories. An example is cannabis as it has depressive, certain stimulant and hallucinogenic properties.

Cannabis as Psychoactive Drugs

Undoubtedly, cannabis is an interesting drug as it does not particularly fit into any one of the psychoactive drug categories including depressants, stimulants and hallucinogens. Rather, cannabis contains mild stimulant effects with the mimic of a depressant. At the same time, it does have some mild hallucinogenic effects. For this reason, cannabis is left out of the traditional groups of psychoactive substances.

The users of cannabis experience a wide range of psychoactive effects, particularly due to the widespread impact of the endocannabinoid system on the human body. Some of the psychoactive effects of cannabis are changes in mood, euphoria, altered perception, relaxation, altered sense of time and space and so on. Even after taking high doses of cannabis, people may experience impaired memory, anxiety/paranoia, visual/auditory illusions and hallucination (due to very high doses).

The different effects on cannabis result in how cannabinoids interact with several parts of the brain. Thankfully, such interactions are just temporary and do not last for more than a few hours.

Other Psychoactive Drugs

Among different types of psychoactive drugs, the most commonly-used one is alcohol as it is considered as the most common form of drinking. Just like cannabis, alcohol can impact the brain as it works as a depressant in the psychoactive drug. It has brain changing substantiality that can alter the personality of a drinker.

Different types of depressant psychoactive drugs lead to loss of balance and stumble in the cerebellum part of brain. The heavy consumption of such depressants, especially alcohol, can shrink and disturb brain tissue affecting the memory and emotional response.

Certain types of psychoactive drugs can increase the risk of serious physical and mental health problems while taking excessive amounts. As a result, people may suffer from high blood pressure, liver disease, heart disease and so on. Even they can raise problems like dementia, anxiety and depression. On the contrary, the restricted use of cannabis can improve the condition of such mental health problems like dementia, anxiety and depression.

However, in certain cases, the use of cannabis has hampered creativity while certain psychoactive drugs like alcohol and tobacco may lead to more influential moments as stimulants.

Remedies for a cannabis overdose

Marijuana is the other name for cannabis. Other names include, pot, grass, weed, dope and MJ. According to the FDA (US Food and Drug Administration), Cannabis is the most abused drug in the US among the younger generation.

It is a recreational and medicinal drug but any excess may cause unpredictable effects. Smoking marijuana causes faster, predictable results. It is a Schedule 1 drug -THC or tetrahydrocannabinol. Huge amounts of the drug are necessary to case an overdose. For a fatal dose, 40,000 times THC would be required. On smoking cannabis, THC enters the bloodstream where it activates the CB1 and CB2 in the body. Any changes in the receptors affects the memory, concentration, sensory and time perception and several other functions of the body.

Ingesting too much cannabis in a short duration can cause intense reactions. When ingested orally, it takes longer to affect the system than when smoked but it is also stronger. It can be scary but there is some hope. The British Journal of Psychiatry provides some solace by saying that a cannabis overdose isn't fatal.

One should be aware of the symptoms of the cannabis overdose that includes shortness of breath, burning of eyes, increased heart rate, lack of mobility, severe paranoia, lack of energy and enthusiasm, extreme dry mouth, sweats, lack of focus, and upset stomach.

A person may experience some of the symptoms and in varying degrees. The effects of overdose may last for half an hour or for several hours. In rare cases, it may last up to ten hours. The symptoms usually go away on their own but if there are complications, seek help from a physician. If medications or alcohol have also been consumed along with the cannabis, seek help.

There are ways to counter the effects of cannabis overdose:

1. **Calm down, relax** – When faced with a cannabis overdose, it may take time for the significance or the enormity of the problem to sink in. The first reaction is always panic. Calm down. It will help you think logically. Fear will only worsen the situation.

2. **Stay away from aggravating factors** – Some people experience a heightening of the effects in bright lights, noisy rooms, crowded places, etc. Move to a room that is cool and quiet. If you want to be alone, go to a room where you can be alone; watch TV or just take time off from other activities.

3. **Deep breathing** – Take deep breaths. This isn't easy and there are videos to help you do it correctly. It relaxes the mind and brings about peacefulness.

4. **Drink fluids** – Drink water or lemon juice regularly. Increase your fluid intake. Herbal tea and milk are other drinks that may help. Watermelon, oranges, strawberries etc. are good for consumption.

5. **Boost your blood sugar** – if you experience low blood sugar due to cannabis, it could be help towards your fight against obesity and Type 2 diabetes. If you

experience swings in blood sugar, it could be related to cannabis. Take a glass of warm water with honey.

Basics Cannabis ingredients

Steps to make Cannabutter

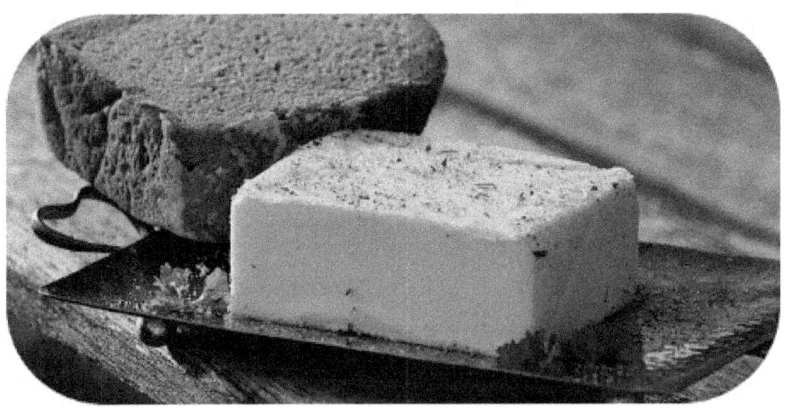

Can you make cannabutter? It may not be too hard to make. By following directions from the experts, you may be able to make the best possible cannabutter in the country. Similar impact of cannabis can be found with this cannabutter. Mild butter is preferred by people on some occasions. The butter can be used with toast. However, you can also use this butter as an ingredient in several recipes. Some baked potato can be added to butter for a great dish. Chopped scallion and bacon pieces can be added on occasion too.

Through strength of the cannabis, the effectiveness of the butter can be decided. By stirring a few spoons of butter into the rum, the taste and aroma of the dish can be changed completely.

Step 1

If you like to make cannabutter like a professional, then it is better to heat the cannabis in a proper manner. Complete activation of THC within the weed can be made possible in the process. It is a kind of technique that is recognized as decarboxylation. For the decarb process of the cannabis, the oven must set to 240°. The cannabis must be spread on the baking sheet in a single layer. Baking the cannabis for about 40 minutes. Even heating can be ensured by turning the weed. Following baking, you may come across crumbly and dry weed. During this time, butter can be added to the tray.

Step 2

On the stove, boil water in a saucepan. It is important to make sure that the marijuana has been lying one inch to ½ inches above the pan at every given occasion. While the water is boiling, butter can be placed on the pan to melt. Minimum four butter sticks must be used for one ounce of marijuana. Therefore, two sticks of butter can be used with a half-ounce weed.

Step 3

Cannabis can be added to the pan once the butter is melted completely. The heat can be turned down now. Cook the weed for almost three hours. The cannabis has been cooked when it looks glossy and water

> **Comment [MB]:** Unclear.

Step 4

Put the finished product in a heatproof bowl but you can also a plastic container. On the top of the container, spread cheese cloth and secure it with tape.

Step 5

Cannabis Butter must be strained now. Spillage must be avoided as much as possible. After straining the butter in the pan, squeeze it from the side for the remaining amount of butter.

Step 6

Cool the Cannabutter for about an hour. Butter can be kept in the fridge until it becomes solid completely.

Step 7

By running a knife over the butter, any water residue can be scraped from the surface completely.

How to make Canna-oil?

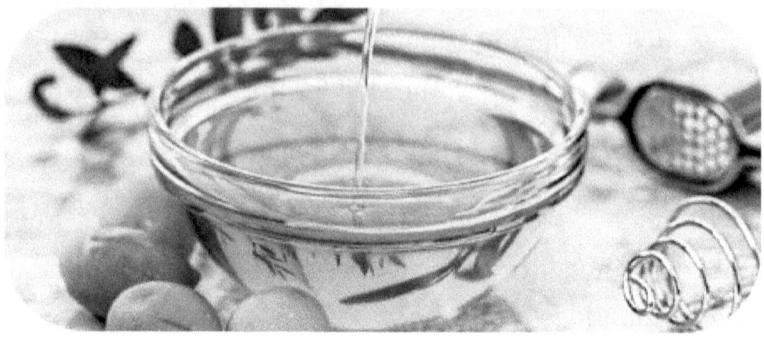

When making choices, try to be health-wise. Health is important to well-being. Physical health as well as mental health are both important. In addition to the food we eat, we need to take other steps to ensure we maintain good health for the long term.

Sugary foods, fat-laden snacks are best avoided. Instead, consider including cannabis infused coconut oil, olive oil to stay healthy.

Since everyone has their own favorites and likes and dislikes, choose a cannabis recipe that you can make part of your life in the long term. In general, create a diet that includes whole grains, nuts and seeds, leafy green vegetables, fruits, lean proteins, eggs. Staying as close to nature as possible when it comes to eating is important so avoid processed food which is artificial, or fake food.

Our food and lifestyle choices very much dictate how healthy we are going to be. The term superfoods was coined to create that group of foods that provide energy, nutrition and boost vitality.

Cannabis is also a superfood in the sense that it provides phytocannabinoids like THC and CBD. Free radicals cause much damage to the body and to counter their ill-effects, we need antioxidants. There are some food items that don't require much planning and time to prepare.

How do you prepare cannabis infused oil? Having canna-oil on hand could be a good way to save time during the weekdays when you need to cook quickly.

Make the oil or butter in advance and store it on your counter or fridge as required. The oil you choose will depend on your preference. Usually, coconut oil, olive oil and canola oil are preferred. Personal preference will take precedence here. Coconut oil is a new addition to many kitchens around the world. Canola oil is mild, and coconut oil has a fragrance that some may not like. Refined coconut oil has no coconut taste.

The important thing to note is that THC will be released into the oil and butter during the boiling process. We don't want to lose it.

When making canna-oil, be care with the proportions. The proportion that works best is one ounce of good weed trim, flower and bud, and 2 cups of oil. The other point to take note of is the two-inch layer of water below the cannabis-oil mixture throughout the cooking process.

Once the oil cools, store it in a container in the fridge and then spoon off the top layer.

Ingredients –

- 2 cups of oil
- 1 ounce of potent marijuana

There are sites that say boiling reduces the potency of cannabis. It is best to keep the heat on low throughout the process. If you need to use the oil for cooking on high heat, use regular oil and use the canna-oil only for cooking items on low heat.

You can also separately fry one item in canna-oil and add that to the dish just before serving.

Drinks

Cannabis Milkshake

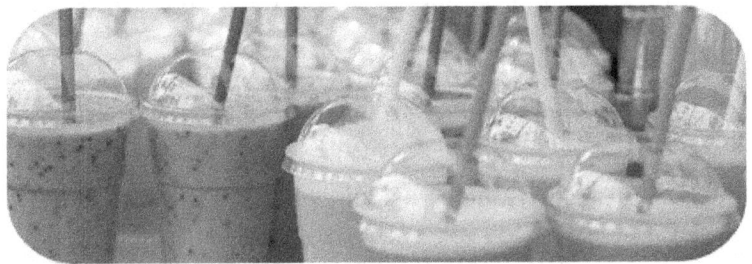

Eating healthy is an important requirement to maintain good health. Bodily health is important to have a long life and stay healthy for longer. Health depends much on what we eat as well as how active we remain.

Eating healthy food is essential since it not only provides us nutrition but also energy to keep going throughout the day. This constitutes consuming food items that do not add to the calorie scale without actually adding to our benefit. Fast food, usually referred to as junk food, is food that does not have any nutritional benefit. Avoiding packaged processed food items, eating the right amount of calories, avoiding sugar and salty foods, etc. are small measures that we can take to remain healthy. Other than eating healthy, exercising is important to lose weight and maintain the ideal weight. Staying fit is a goal for many. Working out for five days a week while also eating right is the best way to stay fit.

We have heard that cannabis can be included in our diet. The herb is required only in small amounts to have the desired effect. It gives energy. To be sure you are on the right track, just keep a handful of the herb in your pantry.

Here's an easy shake recipe for you to make at home.

If you are not lactose intolerant and you like milkshakes, then this recipe could be for you.

Bring out your coffee grinder and grind the cannabis into a fine powder.

Put the milk in a pan and get it boiling. When it starts bubbling, add the fine powder into it slowly. Keep the heat low or else the milk will boil over. This mixture will simmer for an hour. Keep stirring in between to avoid the mixture from sticking to the bottom and the milk from boiling over.

Do not cover the pan or the milk will boil over.

Cool the milk. After it is reasonably cool, **strain the milk** through cheesecloth. If required, strain it twice to ensure there's no sediment at the bottom.

Pour the milk into an airtight container, **add your favorite blended fruits** and store it in the fridge. If you want, you can drink it right away too.

Remember the expiry date of the milk. It's no good wasting food.

Here are the ingredients of this simple recipe.

- 1 cup of milk
- 1/8 cup chopped cannabis
- Strawberries, banana or other fruits.

Increase the amount of milk and the herb if required. Remember that during the hour of boiling, the milk will reduce in quantity. Hence, you may want to add more milk or water as necessary.

Make this simple recipe a part of your lifestyle and food style as it will have good effects. Good things shouldn't wait, right?

Have a Drink with Cannabis Hot Chocolate

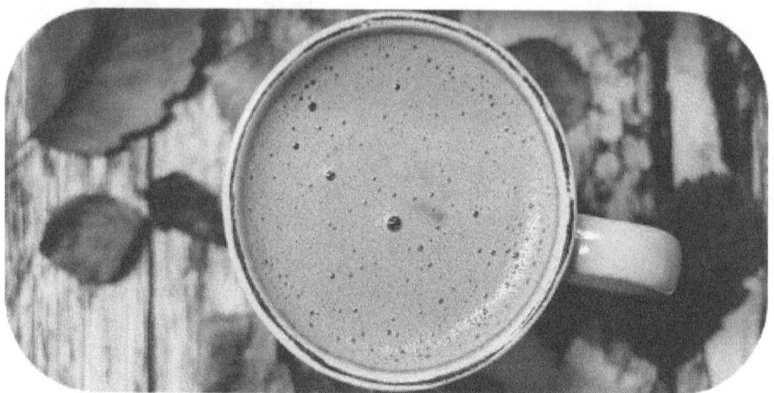

Once again, winter is here, and now is the perfect time to enjoy the coziness of fire while relaxing with some awesomely hot drinks. There is no denying that winter is unimaginable without those hot drinks that can save you from being frozen.

When it comes to hot drinks, why should you try that pine colada mix and traditional hot chocolate again! Now, you have some unique and better options. You can try the all-new medicated hot chocolate drinks. And believe us that once you taste this brew, you can surely get through any blizzard that nature will throw your way. With this hot drink, the cold weather outside becomes much easier to endure. Even if you don't live somewhere where it snows six months in a year, you can still have fun with this cannabis hot chocolate on the colder nights.

Now, getting that warm and cozy feeling for longer in the chilly winter months is not difficult. You must try this recipe as it is super simple, easy and also delicious.

So, are you ready to get the awesome taste of cannabis hot chocolate drink? Follow this exclusive cannabis drink recipe.

Ingredients:

- 1 cup of milk
- 1 cup of water
- 1 teaspoon of butter (here you have the option to use regular butter or cannabis butter as per your choice)
- Hot chocolate mix
- Coffee filter
- 1-2 gm of cannabis weed

Methods:

1. At first, you need to finely grind up the cannabis weed in a grinder. It needs to be mixed well in the water along with milk and the butter.
2. Like other hot chocolate drink preparation, the butter is an important step here. Since THC is not water-soluble, you cannot get as stoned until you add butter into it.
3. Maintain a minimal boil for the water. Of course, you want the hot chocolate drink to be hot, but excessive boiling of the water is not good for THC extraction.
4. Now, let the mixture heat up for around 10 to 15 minutes. When you smell a kind of almond like aroma coming out from the mixture of water/butter/weed, take your favorite coffee mug. Now, pour the hot chocolate mix in it.
5. Take a coffee filter and keep it on the top of the mug and then pour the hot liquid in the mug. It will help to strain out all the cannabis buds from the liquid. Now, stir the chocolate well and enjoy the cannabis hot chocolate in the winter.

6. You can also bring some twist in the drink by adding some whipped cream as well as cinnamon if you prefer. This chocolate drink is enough to keep you high throughout the night due to its intense effect. Hence, you need to plan ahead to stay home in the chilly winter nights.

Meals

How to Make Crispy Cannabis Tacos

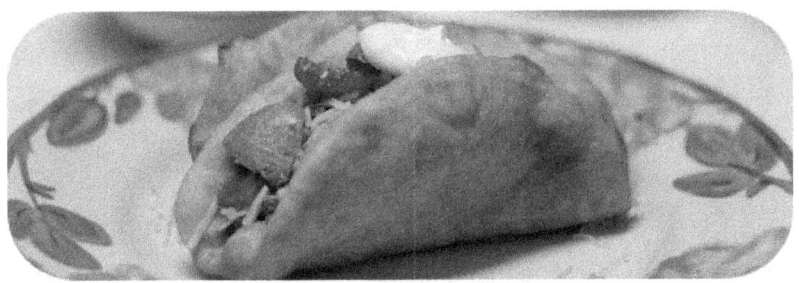

We all love Mexican food as it is thought that the Mexican dishes are the best tasting foods all over the world. Whenever someone mentions Mexican food, the obvious name that comes to mind is the taco, which is a traditional Mexican dish usually made of wheat tortilla or corn rolled or folded around a filling.

There is no denying that food lovers love to experiment with tacos with a wide range of fillings including beef, chicken, pork, vegetables, seafood and cheese to add great versatility and diversity. You have a variety of options for garnishing it with salsa, avocado, chili pepper, cilantro, guacamole, onions, lettuce, and tomatoes and so on.

Now, when you get the chance to indulge in plenty of experiments with tacos, why don't you try something unique yet tasty? Here is a great recipe for cannabis tacos that you will definitely love. Undoubtedly, crispy cannabis tacos is a classic and delicious recipe that you should try; you just can't mess it up. It is truly a delightful treat for your taste buds.

Ingredients

- Ground beef – 1 pound
- Chopped jalapenos or diced green chilies – 3 ounces
- Ground bud of cannabis – 1 to 2 grams
- Head of shredded romaine lettuce – 1 bunch
- Finely chopped tomatoes – 2 pieces
- Taco seasoning mixture – 1 packet
- Water – ½ cup
- Shredded cheddar cheese – 4 ounces
- Salsa
- Small sized diced onion – 1 piece (optional)
- Prepared guacamole – 1 package (optional)
- Crispy taco shells – 1 package

Methods:

1. First, take the ground beef, jalapenos and ground bud and add those ingredients to the skillet. Start cooking until the meat is browned without any trace of pink. Don't forget to drain the fat.

2. Now in that skillet, blend the taco seasoning mix with water and allow it to boil. Make sure that you reduce the flame to a simmer and cook it for 10 minutes. While boiling, you need to stir it occasionally.

3. While the meat is simmering, shred the cheese, shred the lettuce and finely chop the tomatoes. If you prefer to use onions in your cannabis tacos, dice them properly.

4. Check the meat occasionally and when the meat is done, start serving up the tacos. In each taco shell, put a little meat, lettuce, cheese, tomato, guacamole and onion.

5. Now, place the tacos on the plate and enjoy the meal!

Notes:

The delicious recipe of crispy cannabis tacos can be doubled, tripled or even quadrupled. Once you start eating this cannabis recipe, you will find it tough to control yourself. Even if you don't use cannabis, this taco recipe is still delicious and will soon become one of your favorite dishes!

TIP:
If you don't find any taco shells, you can still make a delicious cannabis taco salad following the same recipe.

It's Time to Try a Delicious Cannaburger Recipe

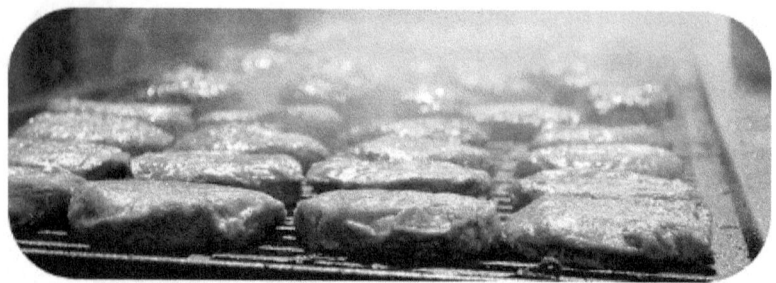

We all love hamburgers. And to be more candid, many of us also like cannabis or marijuana. In fact, few people love cannabis much more than hamburgers. Now, what happens if we combine these two of our favorite things? Cannabis does not always mean you need to smoke it. Therefore, people who don't want to smoke the weed can easily opt for medicated marijuana or cannabis.

So, when we combine a medicated weed with hamburger to prepare the medicated hamburger, it becomes a cannaburger. Doesn't it sound delicious? In fact, the cannaburger recipe is quite simple and delicious and will indeed give you a twist in your taste buds. And if you don't find this delicious, then you need to check the presence of your taste buds.

Those people who don't eat meat may convert the recipe into a vegan or vegetarian burger.

Ingredients:

- Good quality cannabis – roughly 3 to 3.5 grams (it is better to make a fine powder with the ground cannabis)
- Ground beef – 1 lb (the more fat in the meat, the better taste of burger produced)

Note: For the vegetarian burger, you can substitute the beef with different vegetables as per your choice)

- Extra virgin olive oil – 1 teaspoon
- Egg – 1 (for the vegetarian burger, substitute the egg with egg replacer)
- Worcestershire sauce – 1 ½ teaspoon (optional)
- Ground mustard powder – 1 teaspoon (optional)
- Salt and pepper as per your taste

Some other add-ons include – garlic powder or minced garlic, fresh herbs, finely chopped onion of choice, cheese of choice, buns and condiments if you wish.

Methods:

1. First, wash your hands and use them for mixing all the ingredients above into a large bowl. While mixing the ingredients, make sure that cannabis as well as other ingredients are evenly spread throughout the meat.
2. Then the mixture should be formed into patties. Place them on a clean pan or plate until you prepare the other part of this recipe. In the meantime, wash your hands properly as you have handled raw meat.

3. Take a grill and preheat it for the cannabis burger. You can also use a frying pan on a medium high heat.

4. Then place all the patties over the heated surface of the grill or oven and flip once. Make sure that each side is cooked for 4-5 minutes (this duration will depend on your preference). When the burgers have been properly flipped, add a slice of cheese to each one and let it melt.

5. Now, let the burgers cook and in the meantime, prepare the buns and condiments. You can also have optional garnishes along with tomatoes, onions, lettuce and sprouts. Now, garnish your ingredients as per your preference.

6. In this way, you will ultimately prepare the burgers by getting your desired taste. Now place all the burgers onto the prepared buns and garnish them as per your choice.

Now, it's time to enjoy your cannaburger!

Delectable Cannabis Spaghetti Sauce Recipe

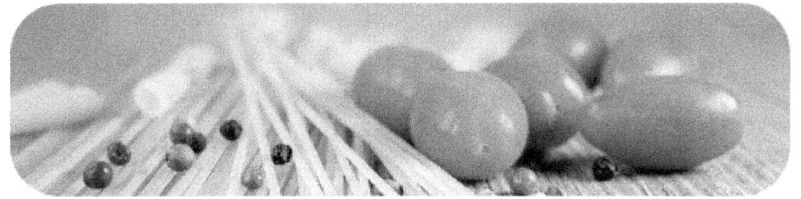

Isn't it a great idea to make an already scrumptious and widely popular dish in better way so that it becomes much more worthy of our cravings? No one can resist the mouth-watering taste of spaghetti sauce. This traditional Italian is considered among one of the most popular staple foods throughout the world. Now, if you want to make the dish more delectable, the best way is to make it with cannabis spaghetti sauce. Simply, you just prepare the infused concoction and add an amount of cannabis as per the level of your tolerance. You can take this cannabis spaghetti sauce with noodles if you like.

Remember that though this recipe sounds unique, it has been concocted and perfected over several years and you vary it with cannabis spaghetti sauce to make it more exclusive and add some personalized flavor.

This recipe is a perfect solution for people who prefer to enjoy legal cannabis, but don't want to smoke it. Like other cannabis recipes, you are going to use cannabis butter or cannabutter as well as cannaoil. However, you need to strictly maintain the amount of these ingredients mentioned to avoid the body from getting too high.

Undoubtedly, the taste of cannabis mixed with the spaghetti tomato sauce definitely creates something that is more suitable to its flavor. After all, the flavor contrast of this cannabis spaghetti sauce is great!

Required Time for the Recipe: 2 hours

Yields 4 to 6 Servings

Ingredients You Need:

- ½ cup of cannabutter
- 2 tablespoons of cannaoil
- ½ finely chopped onion
- 8 oz of canned tomato paste
- ½ cup of purified water
- ½ cup of red pepper, finely chopped
- 1 crushed garlic clove
- ½ teaspoon of pepper
- 1 bay leaf
- ½ teaspoon of salt
- ½ thyme
- One large saucepan

Steps to Follow:

1. Take a large saucepan and mix all the ingredients in it.
2. Now, simmer the mixture for two hours on low heat and don't forget to stir the mixture frequently.
3. After around two hours, the spaghetti sauce is ready with its mouth-watering aroma, serve it over the noodles as per your choice.

There is no denying that cannabis spaghetti sauce recipe sounds easy enough. In fact, it might be one of the easiest recipes that you have ever tried in your life. The great thing is that this amazing spaghetti sauce won't make you disappointed with its burst of flavor as it makes the overall spaghetti high enough.

However, always keep in mind that since you are mixing cannabis in this spaghetti sauce, you should consume it carefully and never consume more than the amount that your body can actually tolerate. When you are going to serve the sauce with spaghetti or any choice of noodles to your guests for dinner, it is advisable to also make some non-infused sauce for your guests with this infused one. Since spaghetti is delicious and some may not prefer to take weed with it, you should have a preferable alternative.

Make Skirt Steak Salad with Cannabis

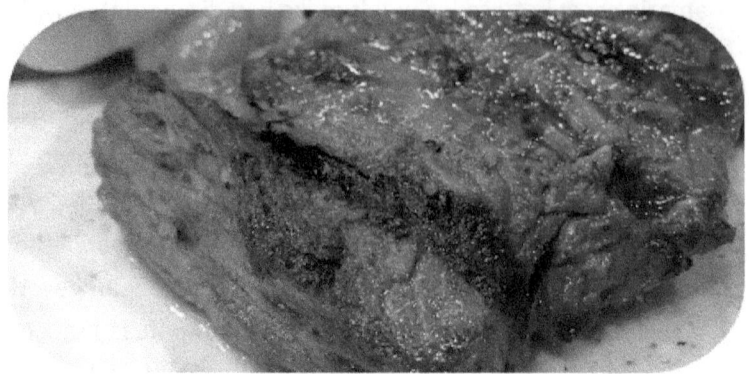

A simple method of cooking can be found with cannabis. Some people believe that you have to be experienced to cook with cannabis which is not true at all. Both drink and food can be made with cannabis.

Cooking recipes with cannabis may be much easier than you have ever thought in your life. Quickly, you can make a cannabis infused recipe. Several ways can be found to incorporate marijuana within a recipe. Lots of flavors can be found in the process. In addition, some therapeutic qualities can also be enjoyed at the same time.

A safer way to consume cannabis can be found through cooking. Interesting menus can be developed with the process. It has been always considered as a healthy alternative to smoking.

Have you been looking for a cannabis recipe? Do you want to try cannabis with skirt steak salad? Grilling meat is one of the best ways to consume it.

Pair steak with citrus flavor. Fresh yet spicy green can be added to the dish also. Instead of green, you may use tofu and chicken as option also. Sweetness can be added to the dish with a little bit of balsamic vinegar.

Previously, bargain cut meat has been used with the steaks. Enough amount of protein can be consumed with the process. Both medium and medium rare meat can be used with this cut. However, it may not be liked by everyone in the world. Toast, ripe tomatoes and peeled garlic and cloves can be used on occasion. Canna olive oil can be drizzled on occasion.

Skirt Steak Salad with Cannabis

Ingredients:

- Skirt Steak (20 ounce)
- Chili powder (1tbsp)
- Lime Juice
- Cilantro (2 brunches)
- Parsley (1 brunch)
- Scallions (1 brunch)
- Arugula (1 brunch)
- Carrot shredded (1/2 cup)
- Cherry Tomatoes (16)
- Canna Olive Oil (2 tbsp)
- Olive Oil (1 tbsp)]
- Balsamic vinegar (3tbsp)
- Dijon mustard (2tsp)
- Salt and pepper

Instructions

Placing the steak on a board or work surface and rub some lime juice over it. Chili powder can be added over it also. Grill until it has reached your desired stage of eating and then rest the steak about 10 minutes.

Cilantro, scallions, parsley, carrots, arugula and tomatoes can be combined within a bowl. In another bowl, mix little bit of canna olive oil, balsamic vinegar and olive oil in addition to mustard. Add pepper and salt to the mix. It is better to serve the steak with greens. A little bit of tossing can be done prior to serving also.

By following the recipe's instructions, you will get an amazing dish without any hassle.

Desserts / Snacks

Recipe for Cannabis Chocolate Chip Cookies

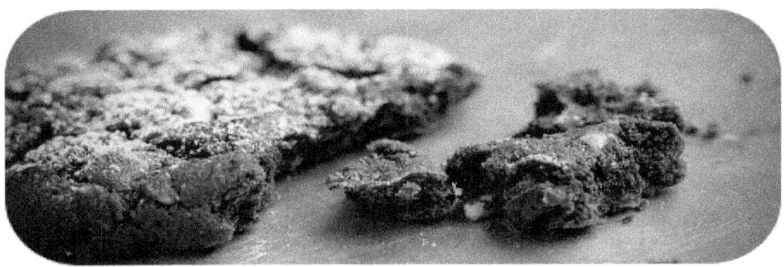

Who doesn't love to eat chocolate chip cookies? But if you are a cookie lover and tired of getting the same taste of chocolate chip cookie, now is the time to make a twist in your taste buds. Why not taste the awesome cannabis chocolate chip cookies!

Well, don't get scared about cannabis if you don't want to smoke it. Actually, consumption of cannabis is quite a good solution for those who don't prefer to smoke cannabis. It is also suggested for those who want to opt for medical use of cannabis. Or you simply want to make some weed cookies and spend the weekend with your friends. Whatever your reason, here's how you can learn how to start cooking with cannabis.

In most cannabis recipes, you need to use a certain amount of cannabutter or canna oil to replace the regular butter or oil.

This cannabis chocolate chip cookie recipe is a great alternative to smoking cannabis or marijuana. So, why don't you try to make your unique cookies using cannabutter! Here cannabis means the edible one as its potency is dictated by the quality of the cannabis.

Ingredients:

- All-purpose flour – 2 cups
- Baking soda – 1 teaspoon
- Cannabis butter (also known as cannabutter) – 1 cup
- Eggs (room temperature) – 2 eggs
- Chocolate chips – 2 cups
- White sugar – ½ cup
- Brown sugar – ½ cup
- Baking soda – 1 teaspoon
- Vanilla extract (good quality) – 1 teaspoon
- Finely chopped nuts – 1 cup (it is optional as if you don't like nuts, you can replace it with some more chocolate chips)
- Salt – 1 teaspoon

Methods:

1. First, take the cannabutter and place it into a bowl.
2. Take another small bowl and mix the flour, salt and baking soda.
3. Now, take the cannabutter bowl and add white sugar and vanilla and mix all of them well.
4. Then, add one egg in the mixture and beat well until it is completely mixed. Now, take another egg and mix it in the same process.
5. Mix the flour mixture from the small bowl into the cannabutter mixture by slowly adding it in the big bowl.

6. Once you find all the ingredients are mixed properly, add chocolate chips and nuts into the mixture and stir well. If you find the dough mix too dry and hard, add small amount of water. Then mix the batter until it comes slightly sticky.

7. Carefully separate the dough mixture into five/six small balls of dough. Now place the dough balls on lightly greased baking sheet.

8. Preheat the oven to 375°.

9. Place this baking tray inside the oven and bake for 10 to 12 minutes, until they are cooked properly. The color of the cookies should be golden brown.

10. Let the cannabis chocolate chip cookies completely cool on a wire rack. Now, they are ready to eat.

How to Make Mouth-Watering Cannabis Dark Chocolate Covered Blueberry Clusters

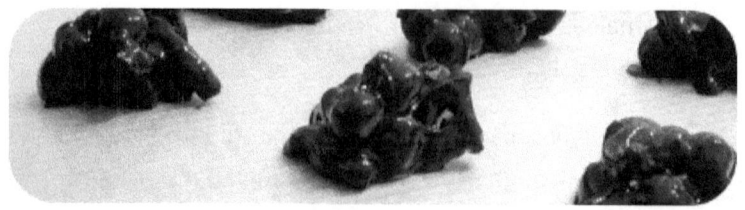

Chocolates are for everyone, for every occasion. Even when there is no such special occasion, you can treat yourself by preparing some special chocolate recipes. And when it comes to chocolate, why don't you choose dark chocolate as it can give numerous health benefits. Now, the question is, how to add dark chocolate during the day?

When you're going to add healthy dark chocolate in your diet, it is always better to get some more health benefits by using cannabis dark chocolate as it has medicated advantage as well. You can take it stony by eating raw or you can get creative with the cannabis dark chocolate recipes.

Here is an awesome cannabis chocolate covered blueberry recipe that you can use as dessert or eat any time to get its health benefits.

Ingredients:

- Cannabis dark chocolate – 1 bar or 1.5 oz
- Properly washed blueberries – ½ - 1 pint
- Curry powder – 1 tablespoon

- Salt – 1 tablespoon
- Medium sized pot along with the lid
- Glass bowl
- Metal bowl or strainer
- Parchment paper

Directions:

1. First, grind the cannabis dark chocolate as finely as possible so that it becomes easier to melt down in the bowl. Now, add some curry powder and salt in the glass bowl and mix them well.
2. Fill up the medium sized pot halfway with water and place a metal bowl or strainer on the top. Ensure that the bowl or strainer tightly fits in the pot and doesn't fall to the bottom of the pot.
3. Boil the water and when it's boiling, reduce the heat to medium heat. Now, put the bowl filled with chocolate inside the strainer and place the lid on the top.
4. Within 5 minutes, stir the chocolate to make sure that it is perfectly melted.
5. When it is completely melted, take out the glass bowl using an oven mitt and put it on a cutting board.
6. Now, take those fresh-looking blueberries and drop them into the bowl by stirring well so that they will be coated all over.

7. Use a fork and divide the clusters of blueberries and put them on the parchment paper.

8. When you have placed all the blueberries on the paper, keep them inside the refrigerator for about 10 minutes to cool down. While waiting, you can also lick the fork and bowl. Or else, you can save the chocolate for other recipes as well!

Health Benefits:

No doubt, the treats of cannabis dark chocolate are quite fancy. The bonus is that these have some great health benefits because of the presence of dark chocolate and cannabis. While dark chocolate is full of nutrients, it is perfect for those who need an energy boost without surplus sugar. Now, blueberries benefit with tons of antioxidants and add extra fruit in your daily diet. Then, this recipe has curry powder that contains turmeric that can give a plethora of health benefits including anti-inflammatory features and potency to fight against cancer cells.

So, are you ready to fall for these delectable cannabis chocolate covered blueberry clusters!

Classic Special Brownies Recipe

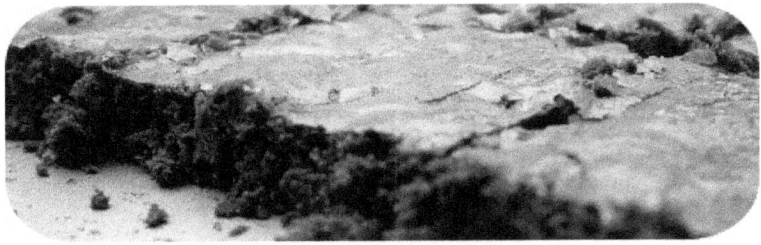

Brownies taste very good, especially when these are taken with coffee. Even the kids love them. The combination of brownie and coffee is just amazing as the sweet flavor of brownie complements the strong flavor of coffee and gives you the wonderful feeling to boost your mood.

Usually, classic brownies are made with a special ingredient in the go-to method and that special ingredient is none other than butter to make the magic. Here, we are going to make a very special kind of brownie – classic special brownie, and instead of using normal butter, we are going to use cannabutter. Nowadays, the cannabis-infused butter is considered as one of the most versatile extractions.

In the classic special brownie recipe, we are going to use this cannabutter to get the job done perfectly well. These brownies are also known as pot brownies because of their special ingredient – cannabutter infused from cannabis or weed. So, these pot brownies or cannabis infused brownies are an edible classic that can definitely delight your taste buds and soothe your mind.

Ingredients

- Cannabutter – 2 tablespoons
- Stick organic butter (unsalted) – 1+2 tablespoons
- Bittersweet chocolate – 4 ounces (Choose Ghirardelli or Baker's chocolate as it can work amazingly!)]
- White sugar – 1 ½ cups
- Cane sugar – ½ cup
- Eggs – 3 (in room temperature)
- Ground Italian espresso – 1 teaspoon
- Good quality vanilla – 1 teaspoon
- All-purpose flour – 1 cup
- Pinch of salt

Directions

1. First, preheat the oven to 350°F (177°C).

2. Take a 13 x 9-inch brownie pan and line with aluminum foil after lightly greasing it.

3. Note: The cannabutter, normal butter and eggs should be at room temperature for half an hour before starting the recipe.

4. Take a double boiler and melt the chocolate on low medium heat. Make sure that all the chocolate is melted.

5. Take the chocolate off the heat and slowly add unsalted butter. Remember that after each addition, you have to whisk the batter to incorporate the butter and make it smooth.

6. When the butter and chocolate are melted perfectly, it's time to add sugar. Then whisk the mixture properly to let the sugar dissolve completely in the chocolate mixture.

7. Now, add cannabutter, eggs, vanilla and pinch of salt and whisk them for two minutes. You can whisk by hand or use a blender on low.

8. Then, take a spatula and add the flour. Blend it well until it is entirely incorporated.

9. **PREFERENCE**: At this point, you can stir in ½ cup toasted/chopped peanuts.

10. Place the smooth batter into the greased and lined brownie pan and let it bake for 35 – 40 minutes. In order to check whether the brownie is done, test it with toothpick which needs to come out clean.

11. **WARNING**: Don't overbake!

12. Now, let the brownie cool down in the pan for minimum half an hour. You can also cool the brownie pan overnight in the refrigerator and then allow it to come to room temperature before serving.

13. Cut into equal pieces as per your requirement and serve with coffee (or hot chocolate).

Nutella high biscuits

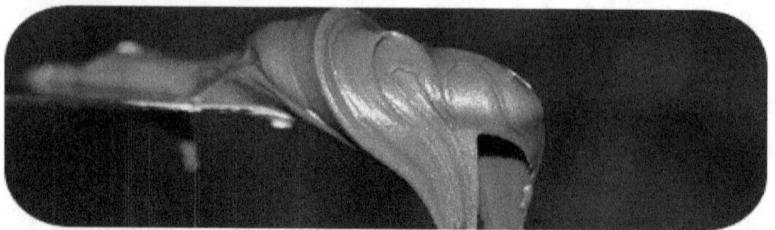

It is easy and requires only a small amount of weed. It is advisable not to change the recipe. Just follow as given.

- Some biscuits/crackers
- Aluminium foil
- Nutella
- Oven

Steps to do it

- Use a small amount of weed say about .2 grams or .4 grams.
- Tear a small bit of aluminium foil and pack the weed in it. Don't double cover it but just wrap the weed sufficiently.
- Pre-heat the oven to 110C (230F).
- Insert the wrapped ball of weed and let it bake for about 15 minutes.
- Meanwhile, take two cookies and spread Nutella thickly onto both sides.

- Now open the foil in which you heated the weed. Sprinkle it over the Nutella. Take a toothpick and spread it evenly over the Nutella. The other way to do it is to take a few spoons of Nutella and mix the herb with it and then apply it over the cookies.

- Now sandwich the two cookies and wrap them in f oil. Put it back into the oven after preheating it to 150C - 302F.

- Leave it there for 20 minutes.

- Take it out and let it cool before you start eating it.

It will take about 45 minutes to an hour or so for the effect to take place. **Don't overeat** if you don't see its effects within this time frame. Once you start feeling high, it will last for about 4-6 hrs.

Give a treat to your taste buds with Frozen Trifle Dessert infused with marijuana

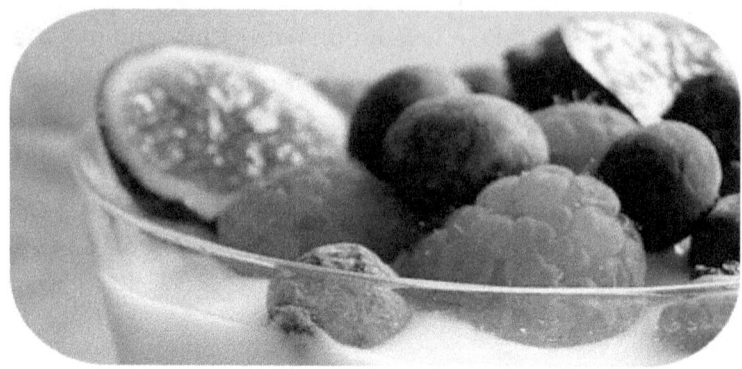

Cannabis recipes can be tried whether you are vegan or non-vegetarian. Delightful dishes can be developed with the assistance of cannabis. Dry fruits or crumbled nuts can be used for these recipes also. Do you like to eat cannabis infused pie crust or creamy avocado? Luscious filling can be made easily with ginger and citrus. The sweetness of the dish can be enjoyed even if you are not using sugar. Processed food must be avoided at any given occasion. Instead, you may try cannabis infused dishes. For an energetic high, coconut oil with cannabis can be tried also.

Fat filled items must not ever be eaten and the pantry must be laden with nutritious food at every given occasion. Potent infusion can also be made from olive oil and coconut oil. A medicated and healthy diet with cannabis can be created in the process. Leafy greens, nuts, grains and seeds are always good for health. Packaged convenience must be eradicated from life for health reasons. Packaged foods can be made quickly. However, it is certainly not good for the body at all.

Through super foods, a necessary boost can be given to the body. Vitality, focus and energy can be added to the life.

Phytocannabinoids such as CBD and THC can be infused within the body by using cannabis properly. Omega 3 and 6 in addition to benefits of amino acids can be found with hemp which is a type of cannabis. Homeostasis of the body can be maintained with the process very naturally. It works towards restoring vitality also.

Some healthy and lovely dessert recipes infused with cannabis can be found that are good for your health as well as your taste buds.

Trifle recipes are loved and adored. For a perfect dessert, trifle can be pitched quite easily. Cakes, custard, fruits and whipped cream can be combined for the creation of a recipe.

A legendary dessert can be made from trifle with three layers. Cannabis can be added to the recipe at the time too. An excellent trifle can be made in the process.

Frozen Trifle Infused with Cannabis

Ingredients:

- Greek vanilla yogurt (16 ounce)
- Cannabutter (2tbs)
- Blueberries (1 ½ cup)
- Honey (2tbs)

- Food cake (1 ½ cup)
- Strawberries (1 ½ cup)

How to make it

First, blend cannabutter, yogurt, honey and blueberries using a blender. 1/3 of the mix must be retained in the freezer for cooling effect.

Put the food cake in four bowls. Place the mixture of 2/3 un-refrigerated blueberries and yogurt in the bowl with the food cake. Then freeze the bowl in the freezer.

A few minutes later, place the strawberries on the top. The remaining part of the blueberry and yogurt mixture must be put on the top. By freezing the bowl, it can be made firm. Later, the trifle must be kept at room temperature.

Cannabis-infused candy recipes that are easy to make

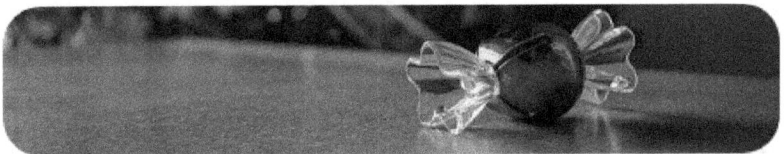

Making cannabis infused food items isn't always easy. That depends on what you intend to make. Some recipes are quite easy to make. Others require perfect measurements and include a long list of ingredients.

Food is an essential part of our life. It creates good health. Eating right is the way to good health. Including cannabis in the diet is the right approach. The item is potent and if taken in the right amount gives energy, or a lot of fun.

There are easy ways to make cannabis-infused candy. The candies are easily available in dispensaries but eating a home-made one is more cost-effective if done regularly.

Canna Gummy

Take out the gummy molds. Buy a box of Jell-o mix. Follow the instructions to make Jello. Add a little cannabis tincture, pour and allow to cool. You can add a bit more cannabis if you want.

Canna Rangers

Here's another simple recipe to make potent candies. You will need a candy thermometer to judge the temperature. Buy a bag of Jolly Ranchers. There are $3 bags in the market. Throw the candies into a coffee grinder. Choose the color you want. Either mix all of them together or separate them based on the color.

Add ¼ cup of water to the ground Jollys and add them to a pan. Put the pan onto the stove and increase the temperature to 300 degrees. Use the candy thermometer.

Once the mixture reaches 300 degrees, switch off the heat. Add the cannabis tincture – as much as you want.

Pour the contents into a mold or onto a cookie sheet covered with non-stick foil. Let it harden.

Cannaghee –based jalebis

Cannaghee –based jalebis are made of flour that is fried in cannabis-infused ghee (Clarified butter). It takes some preparation to make this Indian snack but the result is some delicious, sweet, herbal stuff that will melt in your mouth. The item may be too sweet for everyone to consume in handfuls.

Coconut cannabis covered raisins.

There's the coconut cannabis covered raisins. Take a cup of raisins. In a pan, heat coconut oil, honey and vanilla extract on low heat. Heat all the ingredients until all are mixed well. Put the raisins in a small bowl. Remove the saucepan from the heat and pour the mixture over the raisins.

The raisins should all be covered. Let the bowl sit for ten minutes. Remove the raisins to a wax paper covered baking sheet. Store in the refrigerator for 30 minutes until cooled.

Conclusion

These recipes are simple and easy to make at home. Cannabis has been found to have good effects on the human body if taken in controlled amounts. We have medical evidence to prove the above. Hence, the herb has found a place in the diet everywhere in the world. In every culture, though, it is not part of the everyday diet.

Use cannabis if you are a fan of it. There are other ways of including it in the diet. Canna-infused oil to cook food items that can be cooked in low heat is the easiest way.

Marijuana or cannabis is the same thing. It is consumed the world over for its ability to get people on a high. However, it is to be noted that people get high from smoking it but the weed gives better results when eaten. Oral consumption takes time to show its effects but the effects are stronger.

For an hour or so, there will be no reaction. It starts only later and may last for several hours. Smoking cannabis is illegal but eating it in small quantities might not really land you in prison. But you still may be caught for its possession. Be careful.

If you want intense effects eat cannabis. Find out ways to add it to your everyday stuff. There are numerous ways to do so. Add it to the milk but you will have to boil the milk for an hour or so to get the effect. Drink it immediately or store it in the fridge. Include it in your cookies or brownies. These are everyday things that you eat around the home.

Eating it may be as illegal as smoking it but if you have a cake loaded with cannabis, you are less likely to be caught.

No wonder the US President Clinton never smoked hash.

The other important point to note is that cannabis is required only in small quantities. It otherwise tastes awful.

It will help if you sprinkle the herb evenly over the food you are preparing. Since we are looking for THC to enter our bloodstream, adding it to light foods is the best way otherwise it may take longer for it to enter the bloodstream.

In Asian cooking, there is clarified butter or ghee which is helpful in deriving the benefits of cannabis. Remember not to burn the ghee or oil. Once it melts, add the finely powdered cannabis. Keep the heat low when cooking.

The other important point is to cook several items of the same size to keep the proportion under control. Since you are not measuring the cannabis before sprinkling it, we don't really know how much we have added. One cookie may have more of it while another may have less. That will result in the effect also varying. If you eat one and see nothing even after an hour or so has passed, try eating another. This is not the best way to eat the stuff.

Use chocolate to mix the powdered herb. But be sure to heat it before sprinkling it. Its potency can only be stirred after it is heated. The THC in it remains unaffected otherwise and you may not get the desired high.

Have fun!

Check Out My Other Books

Below, you'll find some of my other popular books that are popular on Amazon and Kindle. Simply click or type on the links below to check them out. Alternatively, you can visit my author page on Amazon to see other work I've done.

- **CANNABIS GROWING:**
  A complete and simple guide on growing (medical) marijuana at home.
  http://amzn.to/2jXSDr2

- **HERBS GARDENING:**
  A complete guide on easily growing herbs at home.
  http://amzn.to/2lfFcHT

If the links do not work, for whatever reason, you can simply search for these titles on the Amazon website to find them.

www.ingramcontent.com/pod-product-compliance
Lightning Source LLC
Chambersburg PA
CBHW070151230526
45471CB00002B/616